Trigeminal Neuralgia:

A natural approach to living pain free

By

Dr. Danielle West-Stellick, N.D.

The information contained in this book is not intended or implied to be a substitute for professional medical advice, diagnosis or treatment. All content, including text, graphics, images and information, contained in this book is intended for general information purposes only. You are encouraged to review all information regarding any medical condition or treatment with your physician.

ISBN: 978-1-887219-42-6
Published in the United States of America

Table of Contents

Dedication

To my husband, a man of incredible insight and amazing patience...

Introduction

Trigeminal Neuralgia. A life changer if ever there was one. Born with what years ago would be called "a poor constitution." I, like many, suffer from numerous chronic illnesses, many of which are quite painful. Over the many years, I just learned to adjust. But – as I said, when Trigeminal Neuralgia hit, **THAT** was the game changer! For the last six (6) years I suffered from Type 1. And then Type 2 also started six (6) months ago.

Also suffering from occipital neuralgia for over 12 years, I watched as my fellow sufferers went from one neurologist to another in search of understanding and a cure. I watched as many downed pharmaceutical after pharmaceutical, often with little relief and overwhelming side effects. I also watched as sought surgical interventions some of which helped, others which did not or only provided temporary solutions.

As a naturopath, I did not rely on pharmaceuticals or surgery for my occipital neuralgia, and it's been under control for the last ten years. Yes, there are days when I think my head and neck will explode, and I might wish it actually happen to end the misery. However, by and large, I am in control and completely functional *and pain free* 99.9% of the time.

And – the exciting thing is that, when the game changer struck, at least for Type 1, I was managing it fairly well. When Type 2 also struck, I was overwhelmed. No other way of saying it. As a doctor, I understood what was happening which made it even more frustrating, knowing that it was time once again to put my naturopathic hat on and help myself.

BUT – here's the encouraging thing I hope to pass on to you all through the pages of this book – within a few days of experimenting to tailor what worked for me, I am one again highly functional and overwhelmed not by disorder or dysfunction, but by healthfulness and wellbeing.

What I am about to share are many of the alternative therapies available for Trigeminal Neuralgia. Not all remedies or modalities work for everyone, just as not all pharmaceuticals or surgical interventions work for everyone the same. While I do not purport to offer a cure, what I do offer is healing, health, and wellbeing free of discomfort. To some that might be a state of remission, to others it's functionality. To all, it is the hope of freedom.

As a naturopath, when I work with any client regarding any illness or type of disorder, I always start with providing the person with a brief education on it. Often, we only half hear what a doctor tells us, or we just know our symptoms and a doctor tells us a diagnosis – but we don't really know what is happening or why. Through a series of brief introductory chapters, I will attempt to help you understand exactly that, what is going on with you and why suddenly it feels like lightning bolts are surging through your face or like you've been hit in the jaw with a 2 X 4. In other words, we'll start with some basic neurology, neuroanatomy, and of course discuss Trigeminal Neuralgia.

Following this, I'll discuss many of the pharmaceutical and surgical options a traditional neurologist or neurosurgeon might offer as a treatment or cure for Trigeminal Neuralgia.

Following these general chapters, the remainder of the book will focus on alternative natural options available emphasizing the supplement route of herbs and homeopathics. Although there are other modalities available that are considered within the natural healing realm, such as massage therapy, reiki, and so forth, personally I a very reticent to endorse these as specific treatments for Trigeminal Neuralgia as it is such a widely misunderstood beast and few practitioners really know what the disorder is in the medical realm. When you get into the allied medical realm where reiki and massage therapy are, and again, this is my personal belief, you need to tread very carefully.

Although this is a book on natural and alternative methods for pain control with Trigeminal Neuralgia, I felt it important to truly understand your disorder including the anatomy and physiology involved; thus, the initial detailing of the early chapters. However, tt is based on the supplement section that I offer help and healing to all, and wish you success!

Now, get ready to read, understand, and move forward on your road to wellness!

Chapter One: Neuroanatomy 101

If you look at the nerve cell (neuron), you can see its basic structure. The roundish image at the center of all the lines shooting off from it is called the somas; it's the actual cell body of the neurons and contains the nucleus. The lines shooting off of the soma are referred to as neurites. There are two types of neurites: dendrites (which are the receptors of the nerve cell, in other words they receive synaptic inputs from other neurons) and axons (which actually conduct nerve impulses).

FUN FACT: Believe it or not, the ability to see the individual nerve cell (neuron) dates back to the late 1890s. As medical science and research continued, based upon the new microscopic ability, work with brain-damaged patients suggested that certain regions of the brain were responsible for certain functions, including the introduction of neural transmitters in the synapses (space between the nerve cells) where the electrical impulses are transmitted from one nerve cell to another along the path of the nerve itself.

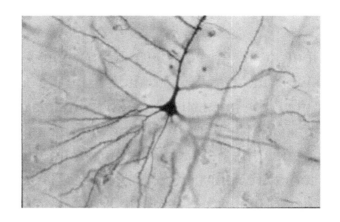

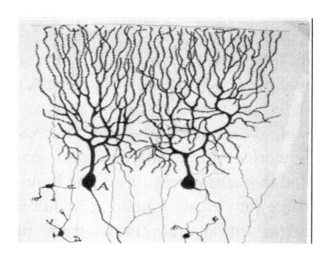

In a nut shell

Neurons are cells specialized for communication. They are able to communicate with neurons and other cell types through specialized junctions called synapses, at which electrical or electrochemical signals can be transmitted from one cell to another. Many neurons extrude a long thin filament of axoplasm called an axon, which may extend to distant parts of the body and are capable of rapidly carrying electrical signals, influencing the activity of other neurons, muscles, or glands at their termination points. ***This is important when looking at such issues as Trigeminal Neuralgia where so many facial and cranial areas are or can be affected.*** Bottom line: A nervous system emerges from the assemblage of neurons that are connected to each other.

Collections of nerve cells come together to form full nerves that run throughout our body; and in most specifically to our interest area, the head. If you think of your nerve system as the electrical system in your house or an electrical appliance, the live electrical wire is your nerve. However, nerves are surrounded by what is referred to as a myelin sheath, much like the coating on an electrical wire. This is of paramount importance in the case of Trigeminal Neuralgia.

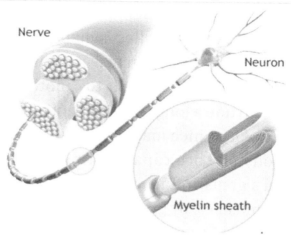

Nerve

Neuron

Myelin sheath

Remember: the nervous system is the most complex organ system in the body, with most of the complexity residing in the brain. The human brain alone contains around one hundred billion neurons and one hundred trillion synapses. The figure below provides a brief overview of why we have so many neurons and associated synapses – they cover the entire body!

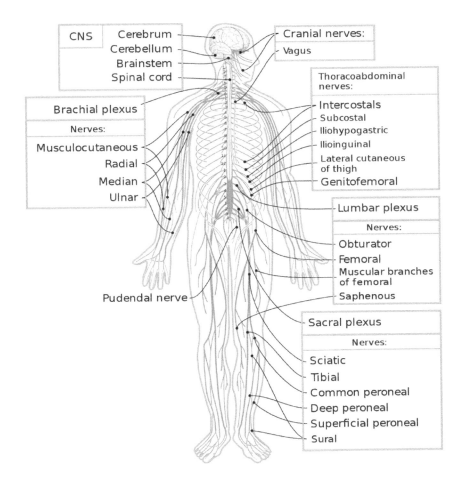

The 12 Cranial Nerves

Continuing with our education on the nervous system and Trigeminal Neuralgia, let's focus on the 12 cranial nerves for a moment. There are 12 cranial nerves in the human body. As we review each of the 12, it is important to note that cranial nerves can transmit two types of information: sensory and/or motor. *Sensory information* refers to those things we associate with our senses: sound, smells, sights, tastes, touch. *Motor information* refers to movements, such as muscle activity. Typically, most of the cranial nerves have only functions related only to one or the other, either sensory or motor, it is important for our discussion on Trigeminal Neuralgia to be aware, some, like the trigeminal nerve, possess functionality for processing both types of information.

It is also important to note, especially for Trigeminal Neuralgia, that cranial nerves come in pairs. One on each side of the head. The following is a very brief description of the function each of the 12 cranial nerves provide

I.   *Olfactory Nerve*: The olfactory nerve is strictly a sensory nerve that provides us with our sense of smell.

II. *Optic nerve*: The optic nerve is also a sensory nerve that provides vision related information to our brain

III.   *Oculomotor nerve*: The oculomotor nerve
        is a motor nerve that is associated with
        the typical movements of the eye, such as
        when you lift your eyelid when you open
        your eyes, rotating or rolling your eyes,
        and even when your pupil constructs
        when exposed to light. construction of
        pupil on the exposure to light and
        operating several eye muscles.

IV.   *Trochlear*: The trochlear nerve is also an
        eye related motor nerve which handles
        the actual full eye movements, such as
        turning the eye.

V.   *Trigeminal*: The trigeminal nerve is
        actually the largest of the 12 cranial
        nerves, is divided into three branches
        (ophthalmic, maxillary, and mandibular)
        and is one of the cranial nerves that
        functions as BOTH a sensory and motor
        nerve. The next chapter will detail the
        vast extent of information that the
        trigeminal nerve is responsible for, and
        thus, for those with Trigeminal Neuralgia,
        why so many areas can be affected.

VI. *Abducent*: The abducent muscle is also an eye related motor nerve that functions in turning the eye laterally.

VII. *Facial*: The facial nerve, as you might imagine, is both a sensory and a motor nerve responsible for our facial expressions as well as supplying the nerve with sensory information related to our face, such as touch and even taste from the tongue.

VIII. *Vestibulocochlear*: The vestibulocochlear nerve is sort of like our gyroscope – although it is both a sensory and motor nerve. It provides information concerned our balance. It also provides information related to our sense or hearing and sound.

IX. *Glossopharyngeal*: The glossopharyngeal nerve is both a sensory and motor nerve that provides information from the upper part of the throat (pharynx) as well as some information from the palate and tongue, such as temperature, pressure, and so forth. The glossopharyngeal nerve also includes sensory information from our taste buds and salivary glands. It also covers some portion of taste buds and salivary glands. The motor functions of glossopharyngeal nerve are responsible for our food swallowing.

X. *Vagus*: The vagus nerve is also a sensory and motor cranial nerve, which is associated with the upper digestive system (pharynx, larynx, esophagus, and trachea). The vagus nerve is also associated with your lungs (the bronchi) as well as some portions of the heart. As a motor nerve, it enables muscles to constrict; as a sensory nerve it helps in our ability to taste.

XI. *Spinal accessory nerve.* The spinal accessory nerve provides information related to most things spinal, such as the spinal cord itself, as well as nearby muscles, such as the trapezius muscle, as well as information related to muscle movement in the neck and shoulders.

XII. *Hypoglossal nerve*: The hypoglossal nerve is a motor nerve that is associated with tongue muscles and movements of the tongue.

Understand, the above review is strictly a very brief discussion to highlight how complex our neck and heads are. While I've documented what each of the 12 cranial nerves are associated with, you can easily see how interrelated each of the 12 are with each other and how much we depend on them in our daily lives.

The trigeminal nerve itself, good ol' fifth Cranial Nerve, is associated with so much, and it is of so much importance to those of us who have Trigeminal Neuralgia, I decided to devote an entire chapter to the trigeminal nerve alone. Only by understanding all of the intricacies of the nerve structure and functions itself can you fully appreciate all that the nerve does for you and where things may go wrong along the way.

Chapter Two: The Trigeminal Nerve

Out of all the 12 cranial nerves, the trigeminal nerve is the largest and most complex. The name trigeminal refers to the three main branches of the nerve: the mandibular nerve (V3), the maxillary nerve (V2), and the ophthalmic nerve (V1). As highlighted in the previous chapter the trigeminal nerve has both sensory and motor functionality, it is primarily divided as follows: the maxillary and ophthalmic nerve provides only sensory functions, whereas the mandibular nerve provides both motor and sensory functions.

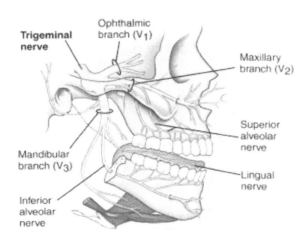

For simplification, the branches are often imaged as pictured below:

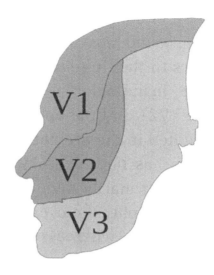

Ophthalmic Nerve

The ophthalmic branch further separates into three branches that carry nerves to:

> - scalp
> - forehead
> - upper parts of the sinuses
> - upper eyelid and associated mucous membranes
> - cornea of the eye
> - bridge of the nose

Maxillary Nerve

The maxillary branch of the trigeminal nerve is further divided into 14 branches that innervate the mucous membrane, skin, and derivatives sinuses of the maxillary area of the face, including:

> ➤ lower eyelid and associated mucous membranes
> ➤ middle part of the sinuses
> ➤ nasal cavity and middle part of the nose
> ➤ cheeks
> ➤ upper lip
> ➤ some of the teeth of the upper jaw and associated mucous membranes
> ➤ roof of the mouth

Mandibular Nerve

The mandibular branch of the trigeminal nerve separates into four branches, bringing nerve functionality to the lower part of the face and head, including

- outer part of the ear
- lower part of the mouth and the associated mucous membranes
- front and middle parts of the tongue
- teeth of the lower jaw and the associated mucous membranes
- lower lip
- chin
- It also stimulates movement of the muscles in the jaw and some of the muscles within the inner ear.

I purposely tried to go into as much detail as possible on the trigeminal nerve, how complex it is, and how much functionality it actually provides while remaining as easy to understand as possible. When we talk about Trigeminal Neuralgia in the next chapter, and the traditional medical approaches to management of the disorder, hopefully you will have a better understanding about why it was important to fully understand all that the trigeminal nerve actually does for you.

Chapter Three: Trigeminal Neuralgia explained and explored

What is Trigeminal Neuralgia? To most, the easy answer is a single word: PAIN! The real answer is much more involved and to be fair, truly takes any volumes of medical texts to explain. However, in this chapter, I'm going to try to take a more general, non-medical, look at what Trigeminal Neuralgia is, for, just as the trigeminal nerve is considered a complex nerve, Trigeminal Neuralgia is a very complex disorder.

What is Trigeminal Neuralgia?

Trigeminal Neuralgia has two forms: traditional Trigeminal Neuralgia (TN1) and atypical Trigeminal Neuralgia (TN2). Although many practitioners only believe in Type 1, ascribing symptoms from Type 2 to other neurological or unknown causes, the difference in symptoms, treatment and expectations is all very different.

Traditional Type 1 Trigeminal Neuralgia (TN1) is a malfunctioning of the trigeminal nerve most often the result of a compression of some type putting pressure on the trigeminal nerve from a blood vessel. This leads to a demyelination of the trigeminal nerve at the site of the compression.

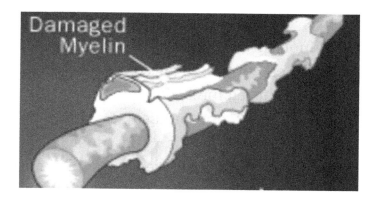

Type 1 symptoms are those most commonly associated with Trigeminal Neuralgia: the electrical shock and stabbing sensation. I've explained it to others as the classic sadist or torturer you see in slasher or horror movies, where the perpetrator hooks up a car battery or generator to battery cables and applies the terminal ends to the victim, shocking them. And then I say, now imagine that as cables being hooked up to an electrified security fence and the terminals being applied to your temple (or whatever area that most affects you) for 30 seconds to several minutes at a time; now you know what Trigeminal Neuralgia feels like.

Type 2 is different. Type 2 does not yield the typical electrical shocks that most associate with Trigeminal Neuralgia. Type 2 is not intermittent like Type 1 pain is, it is constant. Pain with Type 2 Trigeminal Neuralgia can also range from a constant ache to mind-shattering pain.

All the areas of the face and head that the trigeminal nerve affects, as detailed in the previous chapter, can be affected by either Type 1 or Type 2.

What causes Trigeminal Neuralgia?

As mentioned above, typically a neurologist or neurosurgeon seeks to address structural lesions from demyelination. In fact, vascular compression leading to trigeminal nerve demyelination is suggested for Type 1 Trigeminal Neuralgia.

However, in reality, there can be many causes of Trigeminal Neuralgia, in addition to vascular compression, including:

> Trauma to the trigeminal nerve leading, such facial injury, dental injury or a surgical procedure;
> Loss of myelin sheath as result of aging or disease-based condition such as multiple sclerosis (which is why there is such a high correlation between those with MS and those who suffer from Trigeminal Neuralgia).
> Inflammatory disorders like Lyme disease or a host of autoimmune disorders which create inflammation on a systemic (whole body) level, and thus can affect the trigeminal nerve;
> Another class of autoimmune disorders known as collagen disorders, such systemic lupus erythematosus or scleroderma can trigger Trigeminal Neuralgia causes inflammation in the collagen and joints surrounding the trigeminal nerve;

Let me stress, once again – in many cases, no matter how deep you look or try to examine your medical history, there may simply be no specific cause for Trigeminal Neuralgia.

18

How is Trigeminal Neuralgia diagnosed?

One of the most common posts I see in Trigeminal Neuralgia social media groups is that the individual's doctor said "Oh no, you don't have Trigeminal Neuralgia, because..." when the person knows beyond the shadow of a doubt that they do. It's true, not *all* practitioners know the intricacies of Trigeminal Neuralgia, not even neurologists or neurosurgeons. To most doctors they believe the gold standard is a fiesta MRI to pick up compressions – however, as just stated, not all Trigeminal Neuralgia is the result of a compression! And, here's the other kicker: *There is no single laboratory or imaging test that will conclusively indicate Trigeminal Neuralgia.*

However, that said, there are a number of clinical tests that a doctor may perform to assess the nerve itself. For example, to test the sensory abilities of the trigeminal nerve, a doctor may ask you to close your eyes and then will touch your face with a cotton ball in each of the three branch areas. Sensory loss is more typically seen in patients with demyelination disorders, such as multiple sclerosis. To test to motor supply of the trigeminal nerve (and this sounds incredibly painful just thinking about it), a doctor might ask to you clench your teeth; if there is damage to the nerve it will show in the ability to move the jaw from side to side. This usually also happens when the teeth are not aligned.

Few interesting Trigeminal Neuralgia statistics: Given that there is a right and a left trigeminal nerve, the right nerve is affected five times more frequently than patients complaining with left side impairment.

Upwards of 60% of Trigeminal Neuralgia patients experience lower jaw pain from the corner of the mouth to the jaw angle, exhibiting issues with the mandibular branch of the trigeminal nerve, whereas only 30% complain of pain from the upper lip to the eye or eyebrow area of the face exhibiting issues with the ophthalmic and maxillary branches.

Trigeminal Neuralgia typically affects older individuals, however, when the patient already has a demyelination disorder, such as multiple sclerosis, the age of onset for Trigeminal Neuralgia is frequently younger than age 40.

Although anyone with Trigeminal, Occipital, or any other head or neck pain related disorder will bristle at this, given the lack of a single diagnostic test that will conclusively state the person has Trigeminal Neuralgia, because the disorder is ANYTHING BUT a headache, the International Headache Society has come up with the following criteria for a diagnosis:

Primary Trigeminal Neuralgia:
A – Paroxysmal attacks of pain lasting from a fraction of a second to 2 minutes, affecting 1 or more divisions of the trigeminal nerve and fulfilling criteria B and C
B – Pain is described as intense, sharp, superficial or stabbing precipitated from trigger areas or by trigger factors
C – Attacks stereotyped in the individual patient
D – No clinically evident neurologic deficit
E – Not attributed to another disorder

Symptomatic Trigeminal Neuralgia:
The criteria for symptomatic, not primary, are the same, however, whereas primary Trigeminal

Neuralgia, symptomatic Trigeminal Neuralgia not considered as the primary diagnosis primary is related to having a causative lesion, other than vascular compression, demonstrated by special investigations.

Another area that can cause confusion for physicians is the difference between Trigeminal Neuralgia Types 1 and 2. For example, the criteria detailed above relates to Type 1, the electric shock type... Type 2 is very different. Whereas Type 1 is intermittent or random jolts, type 2 can produce constant pain or an ache that covers more area of the face than is typically seen in Type 1.

Given the challenges in diagnosis, often physicians will use treatment regimens as a diagnosis protocol. If the patient responds, a more definitive diagnosis can be made. If not, the physician is less likely to confirm a diagnosis of Trigeminal Neuralgia. The next chapter discusses traditional medical approaches to treat Trigeminal Neuralgia.

Chapter Four: Traditional Medical Treatment Options for TN1 and TN2

Medical Treatment

Traditional medical management in the form of pharmaceuticals for Trigeminal Neuralgia (Type 1) is usually the first thing that will be tried to alleviate the associated symptoms. In fact, pharmaceutical interventions are usually considered adequate for approximately ¾ of Type 1 patients, where patience typically get immediate pain relief with said pharmaceutical use. In addition to side effects which we'll discuss shortly and the toxic nature of pharmaceuticals, the problem is two-fold however:

1) Treatment of Trigeminal Neuralgia must be individualized
2) Relief usually requires greater and greater amounts of the pharmaceutical to continue to alleviate symptoms.

Pharmaceuticals

As a naturopath, I have to state my opinion on pharmaceuticals. Most individuals think that because I look to natural remedies I am anti-pharmaceutical. That is simply not true. There are times when only a pharmaceutical will achieve the results a patient requires for one reason or other, whether it be type of disorder or disease, product availability, criticality of the situation, to assure continued insurance coverage, or even due to financial reasons. If pharmaceuticals can be used as a temporary crutch, that's the ideal situation if the challenge is critical and only a pharmaceutical will provide relief of whatever the situation is. However, if long term use is required, my belief is that quality of the client's life is the most important factor in the decision. Therefore, while this section reviews some of the most common pharmaceuticals prescribed for Trigeminal Neuralgia along with their side effects, please understand, especially as I am a patient with both Type 1 and Type 2, I can fully empathize with you all on the need to reach out for anything that will stop the pain and I stress once again, to me, quality of life is the most important factor!

Let's start our pharmaceutical review with Carbamazepine (also known as Tegretol) is considered the go-to pharmaceutical to use when Trigeminal Neuralgia is suspected or diagnosed. When that doesn't work, second-line pharmaceuticals used are often lamotrigine (Lamictal) is often prescribed for patients with multiple sclerosis.

Carbamazepine (Tegretol) and acts by inhibits neural activity, thus reducing the conductivity of pain sensation. However, use of carbamazepine is associated with many negative side effects including, but not limited to:

- Blurred vision or double vision
- Continuous back-and-forth eye movements
- Changes in normal behavior (typically when administered to children)
- Momentary or longer lasting periods of confusion, agitation, or hostility (typically when administered to the elderly)
- Diarrhea which can be severe
- Feelings of discouragement
- Drooling

- Feelings of fear, unreality, depression, sadness, or feeling empty
- Feeling of reduced interest in normal activities and reduced feelings associated with pleasure
- Feeling detached from the body
- Headache that is constant
- Onset or increase of seizures
- Easily irritated
- Nausea and or poor appetite
- Loss of coordination, poor balance
- Muscle trembling, jerking, stiffness, shakiness
- Shuffling or unsteady walk
- Stiffness of the arms or legs
- Rapid and severe mood swings including mania
- Suicidal thoughts and often attempts
- Fatigue
- Difficulty concentrating or focusing
- Insomnia despite drowsiness
- vomiting (severe)

Interestingly, blurred or double vision or eye movements are known to be more common negative side effects than the others mentioned.

Some side effects of carbamazepine may occur that usually do not need medical attention. These side effects may go away during treatment as your body adjusts to the medicine. Also, your health care professional may be able to tell you about ways to prevent or reduce some of these side effects. It is important to discontinue Tegretol/carbamazepine if you are pregnant.

Lactimil works in a manner similar to Tegretol by reducing neural activity, and thus reducing the perception of pain. The list of common negative side effects is similar to those reviewed above, but not as many of them are considered common. Common side effects include, but are not limited to:

- Blurred vision, double vision, and/or changes in vision and eye movement
- Lack of coordination, feeling unsteady on one's feet and/or unusually clumsy
- Skin rash
- Anxiety
- Chest pain
- Emotional changes including increased irritability, agitation, depression and episode of transient or constant confusion

27

- Onset of seizures
- Prone to infection

Gabapentin has also demonstrated effectiveness in Trigeminal Neuralgia, and is also a pharmaceutical used by patients with multiple sclerosis. Gabapentin works in the same manner as Tegretol and Lamictal by reducing neural activity, thus reducing the sensation of pain.

Most common side effects experienced with Gabapentin include the same issues with eye movements as the previous two pharmaceuticals, however unsteadiness and being unusually clumsy are more commonplace with Gabapentin than the other two.

Other common side effects are similar as well to Tegretol:

- Changes in behavior including increased crying, feeling restless, experiencing agitation and/or aggression
- Emotional changes including increased depression and anxiety, rapid and wide

mood swings, heightened distrust and paranoia, hyperemotionality
- Cognitive challenges including problems focusing and concentrating, memory loss,
- Possessing a false sense of well-being

Physical side effects with Gabapentin also include the possibility of:

- Black, tarry stools
- Fever and chills
- Chest pain and shortness of breath
- Cough
- Pain or swelling in the arms or legs
- Painful or difficult urination
- Sore throat
- Cancer sores in mouth or on lips
- Swollen salivary or cervical lymph glands
- Unusual bleeding or bruising
- Fatigue and muscle weakness

Topamax is also another anticonvulsant, commonly prescribed for patients with Trigeminal Neuralgia. It is also widely prescribed for those with occipital neuralgia and migraines. In addition to common side effects, Topamax comes with major warnings:

- Topamax may cause permanent vision problems
- Topamax can cause severe cases of hyperthermia and decreased sweating leading to dehydration or death
- Suicidal ideations

More common side effects associated with Topomax include but are not limited to:

- Fever
- Weight loss
- Numbness or tingling in your arms and legs;
- Feeling flush
- Increased frequency, duration, and severity of headaches
- Feeling dizziness or un stable
- Feeling tired, or drowsy
- Experiencing slower reaction times
- Fatigue
- Onset or worsening of anxiety
- Onset or worsening of depression

- Onset or worsening of agitation or irritability
- Diarrhea
- Stomach pain
- Loss of appetite
- Nausea and/or vomiting
- Feeling like you have a head cold (stuffy nose, sneezing, sore throat, etc.);
- Changes in your sense of taste.

Topomax must be discontinued if you are pregnant.

Another common mediation prescribed for Trigeminal Neuralgia is baclofen which is a muscle relaxer and an antispasmodic agent. Typically, baclofen is used to treat muscle relate issues including spasm, pain and/or stiffness associated with multiple sclerosis or spinal cord issues.

Typical side effects experienced with baclofen include, but are not limited to:

- Feeling drowsy
- Sense of confusion
- Feeling lightheaded or unstable

- Fatigue
- Insomnia
- Muscle weakness
- Nausea and/or vomiting
- Constipation
- Urinating more often than usual
- Abdominal or stomach pain or discomfort
- Increased frequency, duration, or severity of headaches
- Loss of appetite or change in tastes
- Low blood pressure
- Muscle or joint pain
- Numbness or tingling in hands or feet
- Pounding heartbeat
- Sexual problems in males
- Slurring of speech or other speech related problems
- Feeling like you have a stuffy nose
- Weight gain

Surgery

Surgical treatment is viewed as the next option when relief with pharmaceutical is not forthcoming. In fact, in a recent social media post on a Trigeminal Neuralgia group page, when one individual posted they were at their wits end, that meds weren't working anymore one person commented, "Well, there's always surgery." This is not always true.

With the understanding that the trigeminal nerve is actually located deeper and further away from the surgeon than other access to cranial nerves, Dr. Aaron Cohen-Gadol has come up with the following decision tree flow-chart regarding surgery for Trigeminal Neuralgia that I believe is excellent and provides a very clear picture of what surgical paths, if any, to take.

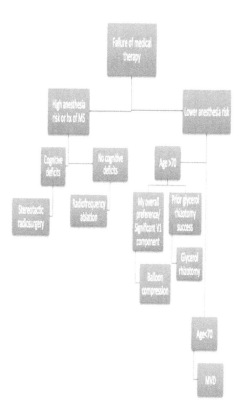

No matter what the situation, the decision to opt for surgery should not be made or taken lightly. It is important to note that all surgery is viewed by the body as a source of trauma. Further, Surgery is generally more helpful in those patients with Trigeminal Neuralgia type 1 where pain is localized, rather than diffuse and as a remedy for the constant pain found in type 2.

Surgery is also seen as a less effective treatment option for Trigeminal Neuralgia in those patients who also have multiple sclerosis or other demyelination disorders.

The good news about surgery for Trigeminal Neuralgia: When successful, upwards of 90% of patients claim that they are free of pain associated with Trigeminal Neuralgia either immediately or very soon after their surgical procedure.

The bad news about surgery for Trigeminal Neuralgia: The pain can return after an initial period of relief frequently requiring either the addition of pharmaceuticals to achieve pain relief, as was the case before the surgery, which may or may not have worked. It is not uncommon either for many patients to require repeat surgical procedures.

It is also considered very important prior to considering any surgery, that all Trigeminal Neuralgia patients should have a fiesta MRI to confirm a compression, and once seen, to rule out other causes leading to the trigeminal nerve being compressed, such as vascular malformations, lesions, or other reasons.

There are a number of surgical options for Trigeminal Neuralgia including: peripheral nerve blocks or ablation, various needle procedures, with the two most well-known and discussed by Trigeminal Neuralgia patients being craniotomy followed by microvascular decompression (MVD), and stereotactic radiosurgery (Gamma Knife®).

Percutaneous Procedures

Percutaneous techniques are most frequently advocated for elderly Trigeminal Neuralgia patients, patients with multiple sclerosis, patients with recurrent pain after MVD, and/or patients with impaired hearing on the other side. Given this approach is the least invasive surgical approach, it is not uncommon for many neurosurgeons to recommend a "needle" approach as the first surgical treatment for their Trigeminal Neuralgia patients.

Percutaneous procedures usually can be performed on an outpatient basis under local or brief general anesthesia at acceptable or minimal risk of morbidity. They commonly are performed in debilitated persons or those older than 65 years. After locating the trigeminal nerve with a contrast material, the contrast material is removed and replaced with a form of glycerol, after which the patient remains still for upwards of two hours to ablate the trigeminal nerve. Balloon micro-compression can also be performed via needle/catheter.

Gamma Knife Surgery

In a nutshell: gamma knife surgery is actually the use of multiple ray high-energy photons concentrated with high accuracy to destroy the specific components of a nerve.

Because radiosurgery is considered one of the least invasive procedure for Trigeminal Neuralgia, it is a good treatment option for patients with co-morbidities, high-risk medical illness, or pain refractory to prior surgical procedures. In fact, Gamma Knife Radiosurgery is the next option after failed pharmaceutical management of Trigeminal Neuralgia if a patient isn't a good candidate for Microvascular

Decompression (MVD) or if the patient is not a good candidate for general anesthesia.

In fact, in a long-term study of 220 patients who had Gamma Knife surgery at the University of Pittsburgh Medical Center, results reported greater than 50% pain relief was achieved post-operatively by upwards of 82.3%.

However, Gamma Knife surgery is not without its risks. The onset of new injury to the trigeminal nerve is possible, as is long-term facial numbness. Typical side effects experienced range from immediate to longer-term. Immediate side effects experienced can include but are not limited to:

Immediate Side Effects

Most immediate side effects are mild and resolve within a few days after you've undergone Gamma Knife treatment. The more common side effects include:

Swelling and Soreness of the Scalp

This is due to the irritation at the points on the scalp where the headframe was secured. In most instances, this will heal up and go away within a few days. If you have sensitive or easily irritated skin, let your surgeon and his or her team know so that they can take measures to minimize potential swelling and discomfort.

Headaches

Many people report having mild-to-moderate headaches following their Gamma Knife radiosurgery treatment. This usually goes away within 24 to 48 hours.

There are a few rare side effects that can happen immediately or within a couple of days of undergoing a gamma knife treatment. These include: reddening or other signs of irritation and inflammation in the area of the treatment, nausea and vomiting, and possibly the onset of seizures. Other side effects that can occur during or following the immediate post-operative phase include hair loss and scalp irritation and pain, localized brain swelling, and potentially facial numbness.

Microvascular Decompression (MVD)

This procedure is commonly performed in younger, healthier patients and has become the most common surgery performed for Trigeminal Neuralgia. Not to be confused with Gamma Knife or percutaneous procedures, MVD is major surgery and requires general anesthesia.

In a nutshell, during MVD, a hole is actually opened in the skull bone in the mastoid area (behind the ear) to expose the typical areas where the trigeminal nerve is usually exposed to compressed or pulsating arteries, and a cushion made of shredded Teflon is placed between the artery/arteries and the trigeminal nerve.

Like any surgical procedure, MVD carries with it the potential for negative side effects including but not limited to: Injury to the surrounding nerves could cause facial numbness, deafness, facial droop, double vision, or difficulty swallowing. There is a risk infection or delayed CSF leak (salt water-like fluid escaping from around the brain and draining through the middle ear into the back of the throat). Patient can temporarily complain of discomfort or numbness around the incision.

Nerve stimulator

Finally, a lesser discussed surgical intervention is the placement of a pain stimulator, especially for those with Trigeminal Neuralgia Type 1. Simply put, electrodes are placed under the skin leading to the trigeminal nerve. Once in place, when the trigeminal nerve "misfires," a corrective current counteracts the painful malfunctioning trigeminal nerve. This is also considered minimally invasive surgery with a very short recovery period.

Chapter Five: Alternative natural approaches - Practitioners

As I stated in the introduction, it is important to understand the origin of your TN to know whether a 'cure' is possible, or just the hope of getting the pain under control or the disorder into a state of remission. In fact, one of the most common misnomers about natural and alternative health options for Trigeminal Neuralgia is, unlike the preconceptions about traditional medicine offering a cure, most believe natural means will not, and are therefore often dismissed before they're explored Another point, just to drive home the issue of getting to the ultimate cause of the Trigeminal Neuralgia – on many of the social media sites, people will say one thing or other, including one surgery or other, worked for them or didn't work for them – and they'll recommend the person they're chatting with discuss this with their neurologist or seek out a neurosurgeon who can help. This is dangerous and can easily lead to dissatisfaction and the perpetuation of misinformation. Whether traditional or natural, not all remedies work for all people the same –

and not all causes of Trigeminal Neuralgia respond to the same treatment protocols as others!

So, that said, let's discuss alternative approaches to the management of Trigeminal Neuralgia.

At the outset, let me briefly explain the difference between the variety of practitioners you might find in the alternative and natural realm for the management of Trigeminal Neuralgia and/or any of a host of other health challenges.

Biological dentist
This is a must for those with Trigeminal Neuralgia. A biological dentist is typically a holistic dentist who has additional training or has done their own research into a variety of challenges that might affect a patient, such as Trigeminal Neuralgia. Most individuals think of biological dentists as strictly those that know how to safely remove amalgam (mercury-based) filling and replace them with composite ones. Typically, a good biological dentist can go far beyond that understanding total health

implications that stem with dentistry. For example, as relates to Trigeminal Neuralgia, cavitations can form where teeth have been removed and bone hasn't filled in properly. This usually happens with wisdom teeth extractions but can happen with other dental extraction sites. One study I read (https://www.curezone.org/dental/dental_ neuralgia.asp) evidenced a 94% improvement following cavitation treatment. A qualified biological dentist will take a 3D panoramic x-ray and be able to identify cavitations and take you through the diagnostics of whether or not they need treatment.

This leads me to another point I want to touch on briefly. My use of the word qualified. I strongly suggest you contact the Face Pain Association for referrals or social media sites for other referrals on qualified biological dentists. One so called biological dentist I went to discussed bone loss at a site of a tooth extraction (not a wisdom tooth), never mentioning the word cavitation. Not three years later, I had another truly qualified biological dentist literally take me on a tour of my panoramic x-ray showing me millimeter by millimeter the levels of density in areas where wisdom teeth had been extracted and cavitations had formed. I had one "excavated" and properly remedied, and along with homeopathic remedies the majority of my Type 2 pain was alleviated.

A qualified biological dentist will also understand the uniqueness of having a patient with Trigeminal Neuralgia when it comes to dental care. For example, if you've had an extraction, you should not have implants if you have Trigeminal Neuralgia. If you have Trigeminal Neuralgia, you should not have your teeth polished or any mechanical scaling or work on your teeth as the vibration will cause a flare. In fact, depending on the patient, you may not be able to have a professional cleaning at all. A regular dentist will not realize these things and shame you; a qualified biological dentist will understand and discuss alternatives that you can practice at home to maintain healthy oral hygiene.

Naturopath

A naturopath utilizes a variety of mechanisms to manage health challenges, be they herbs, homeopathics, naturally occurring substances in the body such as amino acids, diet, reflexology, and a host of other non-prescription modalities to achieve a healthy outcome for their client. A qualified naturopath will work with each patient as an individual, using whatever tools that are in their toolbox to help their client.

Some naturopaths specialize in certain disorders, others do not. Some naturopaths rely strictly on herbs to manage health challenges, others look at a broad spectrum of available remedies. Some carry their own brand of supplements or have their own "storefront," others do not. Personally, I take a more scientific approach, recommending a wide variety of non-pharmaceutical remedies depending on the health history of the individual, and carry only two products that are available on a practitioner only basis for very specific needs (in other words, they're not something you can go to the health food store down the block and purchase) and my fee is strictly what I am charged for them; they do not contribute to my bottom line as many practitioners who sell supplements do.

Naturopaths are doctors and, following a bachelor's degree, and in some cases a master's degree, have completed a four-year and in some places five-year doctoral program. Some states require naturopaths to be licensed, others do not. Any certifications the naturopath might hold should be secondary to their doctoral degree as a naturopath, for example in specialty areas of practice.

Be wary of someone who calls themselves a naturopath who only completed certification programs in holistic health.

Herbalist
As you might suspect by the title, an herbalist is one who typically manages a health challenge with herbs. However, unlike just getting an herb at a health food store, many herbalists pick or purchase their own raw herbs and dry them, encapsulate them or keep them in bulk for teas, and produce their own tinctures, extracts, or teas.

It should be noted that in the US, herbalists are an unregulated area of practice, and they can legally practice their craft without a license or certification. Some herbalist certification courses offer very minimal training, others may require 1600 hours for certification.

Homeopath
As you might suspect by the title, a homeopath is one who typically manages a health challenge with homeopathics. However, unlike just getting a homeopathic remedy at a health food store, many homeopaths pick or purchase their own remedies in a raw state and create their own pellets or tinctures, or homeopathic combinations in pellet or tincture form.

Homeopathic education runs the gamut from certification courses you can enroll in with a GED and no college to 4-year post graduate medical training as a homeopath. Unfortunately, requirements for practice vary considerably throughout the world, and even within the United States depending on where the homeopath received their schooling, professional affiliations, and to be honest, their level of interest in practicing their craft professionally or only for self-care.

Other alternative practitioners who patients mention have helped them through their Trigeminal Neuralgia pain including those who practice chiropractic, Chinese Medicine, acupuncturists, reflexologists, massage therapists, and probably others.

The key to a successful natural approach, similar to the traditional allopathic approach, is it may require the input of several practitioners and modalities to achieve remission or simply alleviate pain. But it can be done!

Chapter Six: Alterative natural approaches – Supplements

Supplements are an essential for the natural approach to dealing with your Trigeminal Neuralgia. These are typically what you'd find going into a health food store and wandering through the supplement section, although some are not as readily available at brick and mortar locations, and require online purchasing, or having a store special order a remedy for you.

This chapter will focus on the traditional remedies specifically used for Trigeminal Neuralgia, although some listed are included as known providers of general pain relief. You'll also note that I have these all listed as individual remedies rather than some of the pain relief and inflammation relief combination supplements available in the marketplace. I like to know what is and is not effective in what I recommend to a client as well as in what I personally take. Additionally, even if it's an herbal combination supplement, everything has an impact on you, including contraindications of one or more non-essential ingredients, or it may even be a non-essential ingredient that you do not tolerate well. I prefer to stick with what I refer to as isolates to avoid these issues.

The following is a general list of the common types of remedies. The herbs and homeopathics listed are provided in alphabetical order, not necessarily as a list in order of most effective. The reason for this is alternative remedies are much like prescriptions – what works for one may not work for another. In my practice and personally, I've seen different people respond to different herbs and homeopathic remedies differently from each other.

Herbs

Quite simply put, herbs are generally plants that are valued for their specific strengthening/ tonifying properties. Most are either dehydrated and encapsulated or put into a solution (generally alcohol) from which to make an extract. I've also made extracts with water for personal use. Please note, herbs carry with them many contraindications, much like pharmaceuticals, and should be used with caution (even though all you want is for the pain to go away, I understand, but you don't want to create another harmful situation while thinking you're safely relieving another)

Blue Vervain as an herb that calms or strengthens nerves. However, caution should be taken when thinking of taking his herb as it can interfere with standard (and other herbal) medications taken for blood pressure regulations and when on mediation for hormones therapy. Large doses will also produce digestive issues including diarrhea and vomiting.

Jamaican Dogwood also works for facial nerve pain and other neuralgias. As an herb that slows the central nervous system, it should be used with caution as in general, the herb is considered poisonous. Minute doses are helpful for facial pain. However, it is not considered safe in any amount for those who are pregnant or nursing or those taking any form of sedative or anti-anxiety medication (whether herbal or pharmaceutical).

Passion Flower is a powerful nerve restorer and

calmer, and is especially effective for help in stress headaches and also muscular tension. While a great herb, like the others here, it is not safe for those who are pregnant, as in this case, it can cause the uterus to contract. It is also particularly important for those with Trigeminal Neuralgia who are considering or scheduled for surgery – Passion Flower may anesthetic effects during surgery and after as well as other medications specifically used on or near the brain and major nerves of the head/face. Therefore, if you are considering Passion Flower as you are getting close to your scheduled surgical procedure, it is important to stop taking it at least 2 weeks prior to your surgery to allow it to clear out of your system.

Other general herbal pain relievers include:

California Poppy, which is a mild pain reliever and can be good for pain or even nervous agitation. Like Passion Flower, however, it is important to stop using California Poppy at least 2 weeks prior to any surgery, as it can have an impact on anesthesia. Another major caution is for people taking prescription sedatives, particularly those classified as benzodiazepine medications, such as Klonopin (clonazepam) (Klonopin), Valium (diazepam), Ativan (lorazepam) and many others. When in doubt, consult your pharmacist; but personally, much as I enjoy the benefits of this herb, I'd not recommend taking anything that affects the central nervous system (other than combining it with Corydalis, see below) if you're going to take California Poppy.

Corydalis is also a pain reliever, primarily for muscles, but I have found it excellent for Trigeminal Neuralgia pain relief, especially when taken with California Poppy. Like all herbs, there are contraindications, for example corydalis should not be ingested while pregnant or nursing; and just as important is the fact that this herb is never used alone but in combination with other herbs or occasionally homeopathics. As stated above, I personally combine this with California Poppy.

Wood Betony, often only referred to simply as *Betony*, is a lesser known herb that can be used for pain, and accompanying inflammation.

Although contraindications aren't as extreme as the for other herbs in this section, the most common negative side effect is digestive irritation.

Cell Salts
Cell Salts are similar to homeopathics, and essentially you make your own solutions. To make a cell salt solution, put up to 10 tablets of each cell salt in a 16- to 24-ounce bottle; fill with water and swirl to dissolve tablets. Sip throughout the day. The two most effective for Trigeminal Neuralgia are:

#6 Kali phos 6X – feeds nerves to provide restoration
#8 Mag phos 6X – used for nerve pain, particularly the shooting pains accompanying Type 1 Trigeminal Neuralgia.

Homeopathics
The choice of what homeopathic to use is based not only on the type of symptom relief it provides, but on the varied symptoms that people are experiencing. For example, some Trigeminal Nerve patients experience pain on

the left side of their face, some on the right. For some it's the Type 1 stabbing pain, for others it's the ache of Type 2. Therefore, I've tried to include these characteristics when noted.

As you can see, the list of potential homeopathic remedies is quite extensive, especially compared to the list of traditional herbal supplements for use when a personal has Trigeminal Neuralgia. Personally, I prefer homeopathics as there is less risk to the person than when using herbs, plus there is greater specificity of when to use a particular homeopathic preparation than with herbs which tend to be more general in nature. Additionally, if the body does not need the remedy taken, it is passed the system through without absorption. In other words, no harm-no foul. Thus, although some may disagree, this section does not go into the same degree of contraindications as I did for herbs.

Aconite is a remedy used for Trigeminal Neuralgia very often used when a trigger for pain is cold dry wind or exposure to cold dry air. Aconite is a great remedy when this is the case, and if primarily affects the left Trigeminal Nerve, although it could affect both, but pain is worse on the left side of the face.

Aranea Diadema is a wonderful homeopathic remedy for Trigeminal Neuralgia especially when the patient experiences worse neuralgic pains in damp or cold weather/climates. Aranea diadema is most effective as a homeopathic remedy for those with Type 1 Trigeminal Neuralgia. Other characteristics you might experience leading you to want to use Aranea Diadema is if your Trigeminal Neuralgia pain is on the right side of your face, particularly effecting the teeth at night immediately after lying down, or when you might feel there is a sense of swelling in the teeth/jaw when you know there is none.

Cedron is a homeopathic that is particularly effective for Trigeminal Neuralgia, especially if you notice your pain occurring periodically at the same time everyday affecting the first division of the trigeminal nerve causing pains across the forehead and around the eyes. This is especially effective as well when the Trigeminal

Neuralgia patient experiences intense pain that is worse in open air and worse after sleep.

Chelidonium Majus is a good homeopathic remedy when Trigeminal Neuralgia leads to major head pain and right-sided migraine like headaches, primarily affecting the first or second branch of the trigeminal nerves. In addition to head pain, Chelidonium Majus is useful when you feel pressure in the eye orbit.

Cinchona Officinalis is often used as a homeopathic remedy for the treatment of neuralgic pain that is constant or recurring every alternate day and symptoms getting invariably worse at night. Pains are worse from touch, draft of air and from jerky movements (sound familiar?).

Colocynth is a remedy ideally suited for Type 1 Trigeminal Neuralgia where electric like shocks are prevalent, primarily affecting the left side of the face and sometimes the neck.

Hecla Lava is a lesser known homeopathic remedy usually used for nerve pain from dental challenges. However, I am including it here as often dental problems such as extractions or decay trigger Trigeminal Neuralgia flares. In this case, Hecla Lava is a perfect homeopathic remedy.

Hypericum is a highly recommended homeopathic remedy for Type 1 Trigeminal Neuralgia, particularly when the disorder onset follows an injury or trauma to the Trigeminal Nerve, with the sensation of a toothache.

Magnesia Phosphorica, like traditional magnesium in mineral supplement form, is also considered a good homeopathic remedy for pain control, and in particular for the supra or infra-orbital trigeminal facial nerve pain, particularly on the right side, for Trigeminal Neuralgia. For those who have Trigeminal Neuralgia triggered by or limiting the ability to open the mouth, Magnesia Phosphorica is also a good remedy to use for the disorder. While a good overall remedy for Trigeminal Neuralgia, it is particularly effective for the electrical-like jolts experienced in Type 1, and characteristically when affected by cold air and pain that is relieved by warm compresses.

Mezereum is a good homeopathic remedy for Trigeminal Neuralgia affecting the left-sided where pain is experienced from the teeth to the ear, but can affect other areas as well. Mezereum is specifically recommended when pain is alleviated with the use of warm compresses and is worse when eating.

Plantago has a marked action upon the inferior maxillary branch of the trigeminal nerve especially when nerve pain affects the lower jaw, often extending to the ear. Plantago is especially well suited for Type 1 Trigeminal Neuralgia.

Platina is a homeopathic remedy for issues that primarily nervous system, and has a special affinity for the Trigeminal nerve. Platina is good for those who experience coldness and numbness of the face, the sensation as if your face is being squeezed in a vise, for an oversensitive state of mind and nerves, and when your Trigeminal Neuralgia pains come gradually and go gradually.

Spigelia markedly affects the nervous system, particularly the left Trigeminal nerve affecting all three branches of the nerve resulting in pain in the teeth, jaws, eyes, temple, bridge of the nose, etc. For those whose Trigeminal Neuralgia is also triggered by cold rainy days, spigelia is a good remedy to use.

The affected area becomes highly sensitive to touch.

Staphysagria is one of the most frequently used medicines for Trigeminal Neuralgia.

Syphillinum is frequently used in the homeopathic treatment of Trigeminal Neuralgia. Severe, violent, sharp pains characterize this remedy, making it a good option for Type 1 pain relief.

Sanguinaria Canadensis is a homeopathic remedy for patients where their Trigeminal Neuralgia predominantly affects the right side of their face, particularly with accompanying symptoms of redness and burning of the cheeks.

Verbascum is considered a good overall homeopathic remedy for Trigeminal Neuralgia as it specifically targets the third branch of the Trigeminal Nerve on the left side of the face in the cheeks and or in the general area of the temporo-maxillary joint, however, you might experience pressure on the entire left side of your face and head. Other common indicators are Trigeminal Neuralgia pain that strikes when there is a change in the weather or even while eating where pain might affect the right temporal area.

Homeopathics are best used to alleviate symptoms when they occur, rather than on an ongoing basis (unless the pain is unrelenting and chronic in nature). Also, for some, symptoms may vary from flare to flare, particularly for those with Type 1 and Type 2 Trigeminal Neuralgia and/or who are affected on both sides of the face rather than one. Therefore, my best suggestion when it comes to homeopathics is to examine the above list and see which most closely match you and your symptoms. If your Trigeminal Neuralgia pain always affects only one side and one facial/cranial area, and only one homeopathic seems to match, there is no guess work. Otherwise, if you suffer from varying Type 1 and Type 2 days, along with sometimes the left and sometimes the right Trigeminal Nerve is affected, get yourself a collection of homeopathics which match your varying symptoms, and keep your list of when to take what handy.

Two last supplements
Although I mentioned I prefer herbs or homeopathic remedies that are in their isolated form, I'm just going to talk about one combination: a combination of *Alpha Lipoic Acid (ALA) and Acetyl-L-Carnitine.* You'll note that this is the only combination I'm recommending, and for purity purposes you can purchase each separately but you can readily find this as a combination supplement with just these two ingredients. Research from several Russian medical laboratories has demonstrated the effectiveness of this combination in slowing down and in *some* cases repairing demyelination by rebuilding the myelin sheath. Therefore, if your Trigeminal Neuralgia is due to

demyelination, this will be of help in slowing the progression down and potentially mitigating the need for surgery. There are no promises with this combination, just as there are none from surgery or other pharmaceuticals, but it is worth including in this book.

The other supplement I want to discuss very briefly is CBD oil. As you may know from the hype surrounding CBD, for most commercially available products, it is from the hemp/marijuana plant, where the psychoactive ingredient, THC, has been removed. CBD oil comes in a variety of strengths as well as a wide of forms ranging from moisturizers and lotions to pills and oils. It is also rather pricey.

Many people swear by CBD for both its calmative and pain-relieving effects, however, much like all pharmaceuticals, herbs, homeopathics, and other options, results depend entirely on the individual. For example, I've tried a variety of CBD strengths in oil and pill form from varied manufacturers, and found zero effect. I've also tried two different forms of a roll-on of the oil, same thing, no relief (although the scent one of the roll-ons was mixed with, it did have a slightly calming effect for me).

My bottom line on CBD is, although it may work for some, it may not for others. Should you try it? That's entirely up to you. I'll admit when your friend tells you how much it helped her fibromyalgia, for example, it's very tempting.

Chapter Seven: Putting it all together

This book has provided a comprehensive background to Trigeminal Neuralgia, beginning with an explanation of the nervous system, facial nerves, trigeminal nerves, and finally a detailed explanation of Trigeminal Neuralgia. Following this, a discussion of various traditional medical options and alternatives was provided. I felt it important to discuss these for the following reason: When faced with a new health challenge, or diagnosis, they turn to the Internet and to social media. Most people will see the traditional allopathic medical options such as various pharmaceuticals and surgeries that others take or have taken, what works for them and what hasn't.

They don't hear or see the natural alternatives or understand how they work. They seek help and options from individuals in social media groups, such as Facebook, who are not necessarily qualified to discuss anything other than their own experiences based upon allopathic interventions and will tend to poo-poo natural alternatives proclaiming they are not cures.

Well, here's an interesting fact: According to the FDA, natural supplements are NOT allowed to state they are cures. In fact, if that word, "cure," appears anywhere on the product label or product literature, there is a very hefty fine placed upon the organization, items are pulled from store shelves, and the company can be shut down.

Additionally, without knowing the cause of your Trigeminal Neuralgia suddenly strangers believe they are the experts at recommending a solution for you, and sadly, many in this situation take that interchange as gospel. I liken this to going into a health food store and asking for a remedy from a clerk who used to be a furniture salesperson or cashier at a grocery store and who knows nothing about your health history. That is like expecting to be able to call a traditional doctor whose name you picked at random from the phone book, saying you want an antibiotic, and expecting a prescription be given without seeing the doctor for an examination, cultures and other blood tests, and a full health history. It doesn't work that way.

Whether in the traditional allopathic or natural holistic realm, what works for one person may not always work for another with the same issues. Every one of us was created as a unique individual.

Okay, off my soap box.

I can tell you from my own experiences as a patient with Trigeminal Neuralgia, and other related and non-related health issues, and as a healthcare practitioner – if you understand the role that supplements and homeopathics can play in your life, even if it seems cumbersome at times, your life can be much more manageable.

Focusing on my Trigeminal Neuralgia:
- When it first hit, was my first instinct to go to a neurologist who would make the electrical shocks stop? Of course.

- Did I recognize my Type 1 as a game changer in my life? Of course.

- Did I reduce or eliminate the Type 1 shocks? Yes, down to almost 1 every few months using natural methods.

- When Type 2 hit, did I recognize that as the most intense pain a human can feel? Of course – there were no words to describe it.

- Am I pain-free 24/7 now? Most days.

- Is your Type 2 pain more discomfort or pain now? It varies, there are still times when on a scale of 1 – 10 with 10 being the worst, I'm maybe at a 2 or 3; most days if there are issues what I feel is really more discomfort and certainly not pain.

- Do I have break-through pain? Sure.

- Do I still cause myself flares? Of course, taco shells do it for me (pout).

- Do I manage the pain and inflammation with pharmaceuticals? Nope

- Have I felt the need to see a neurologist or neurosurgeon? During the initial disease onset, I'll admit it crossed my mind, but I challenged myself as a naturopath to find a solution.

- Do I manage the pain and inflammation with supplements and homeopathics? Yes.

- Do I feel I live a surprisingly comfortable life with Trigeminal Neuralgia? Absolutely.

As I said, we are all unique individuals. How we perceive pain and discomfort varies from person to person. For example, my husband hardly feels any pain no matter how extreme the pain might be, his other senses are just as low on the perception scale.

I am the complete opposite. I have a sensory modulation issue where I experience everything from sensory data such as smell or taste to touch and so forth much more acutely than the average person. This also includes my perception of pain. Where it might be discomfort for one person, or my husband may not even notice it, I am ready to pull my hair out. So, the answers I provided above are probably even more telling on how effective natural remedies and alternative medicine can be for Trigeminal Neuralgia.

That said, do I baby myself as well? Of course. For example, I avoid cold air on my face, I don't talk for hours on end (or I know I'll experience Type 2 pain on my lower left side of my jaw). I take the necessary precautions similar to most of us who have Trigeminal Neuralgia.

However, that said – is it possible to utilize a natural approach to manage and maintain a pain-free life with Trigeminal Neuralgia? Absolutely!

Opening the book was your first step to achieving such a lifestyle. The second step was reading through this book. Now, it's time to take your third step, and the most important one, to sort through the information, make your notes and embark on your own journey towards a pain-free lifestyle and management of your Trigeminal Neuralgia.

Appendix A: Pain Information

Having the answers to these questions will help you clearly detail your pain issues and speed a more accurate diagnosis of your Trigeminal Neuralgia once you find the right practitioner for you.

Where is the pain usually located?

Is it Type 1 Pain (electric shock), or Type 2 (an ache)?

How often does the pain last?

How frequently do you experience pain?

Does anything in particular seem to precipitate or cause a flare?

If you had to paint or draw a picture of the pain, how and where it affects you, etc – what would it look like?

Appendix B: What I've Done to Alleviate Pain

Most practitioners will ask you what you've done so far to help alleviate the pain. Your answers (successes and failures) will help guide them to a more accurate diagnosis.

Medications and results?

Hot or cold compresses and results?

Hot shower and results?

Sleep?

Dark room?

Appendix C: Doctors' Exam, Reports, and Imaging

What doctors have you seen for your Trigeminal Neuralgia (or suspected Trigeminal Neuralgia if not diagnosed yet or at the time you saw them)? What was the result? What did they say the problem was?

Do you have copies of the doctors' reports?

What diagnostic imaging procedures or other laboratory work was performed to help guide a diagnosis of Trigeminal Neuralgia? What did the imaging reveal? Do you have copies of the radiologists' reports?

Appendix D: Herbs

What herbs or other non-homeopathic supplements have you tried to alleviate the pain and discomfort of your Trigeminal Neuralgia?

How much, and when did you take the herb or other non-homeopathic supplement?

What was the result?

Appendix E: Homeopathics

What homeopathic remedies have you tried to remediate the pain and discomfort of your Trigeminal Neuralgia?

How much, and when did you take the homeopathic remedy?

What was the result?

Based on the homeopathic remedy information provided in this book, what homeopathics should you try based on which set of symptoms that you experience?

Appendix F: My Medical Background

What additional medical information about you, as a unique individual, is worth noting for other doctors to know about you?

What other diagnoses have been made and when?

Have you had any surgeries?

In particular, have you had any surgeries to the face, spine, neck, or head?

Have you had any dental surgery?

Have you had any dental procedures, including crowns, implants, root canals, or extractions?

Have you ever been in an accident where there was trauma to the head, neck, face, spine, or face?

Additional notes:

About the Author

Dr. West-Stellick is a much sought-after naturopath with clients literally throughout the world. When not working directly with clients, Dr. West is a well - respected writer, lecturer, and seminar leader.

After spending upwards of 30 years in corporate America in a variety of management positions, Dr. West-Stellick's passion for medicine overcame her business success and she received a doctorate of natural healthcare, establishing and maintaining a very successful practice for 17 years, subsequently spending another 10 years as a medical ghostwriter and researcher. Dr. West is the author of over 25 books on a wide variety of topics, for both the secular and Christian market, including: *Ten Essential and Simple Steps to Managing Your Doctor: Empowering you, the Patient; Authentic, Inspired, Inerrant, and True; In Sickness and in Health; God, Marriage, and Illness; The God Prescription; Fear of Forgetting Jesus; Remembering HIM Despite Dementia; My Life, My Memories; Preventing Dementia Naturally: Assuring the healthy child, adult, and senior throughout the generations; Paleo Basics: A delicious guide to what Paleo is all about, and how to become a Paleo Pro in no time!, and Paleo-licious Pasta: The definitive Paleo Pasta cookbook.*

Other Lariat Publishing Books by Dr. Danielle West-Stellick

Ten Essential and Simple Steps to Managing Your Doctor: Empowering you, the Patient
Ten Essential and Simple Steps to Managing your Doctor: Empowering You, the Patient provides a wealth of information in easy to follow segments that will transition you from being the passive patient to the empowered patient, from waiting and being at the mercy of the medical system to the patient who takes responsibility for their healthcare and their life as they seek to form a partnership with their physician. The Ten Essential and Simple Steps to Managing Your Doctor: Empowering You, the Patient is written in an easy to follow workbook format, including pages you can scan or photocopy and use as is or adapt for your own use. For other situations discussed, such as reaching your physician when you have questions or even emergency situations and need to speak with him, sample scenarios are written out in script fashion, providing the framework for your own adaptation to your specific situations as needed. ISBN: 978-1887219211

Authentic, Inspired, Inerrant, and True
From the beginning, Satan has attempted to make us question God's Word to us. Part of Satan's plan is to cause us to doubt that the Bible is God's authentic, inspired, inerrant and true message to us all. It's easier to look at the Bible as a storybook or piece of literature rather than know God's Word is the truth. Thus, many people think of the Bible as a storybook of a book of historical

literature - therefore, whether it is true or not is immaterial. Many people say they believe in parts of the Bible, but not others. We know that the Bible is authentic, inspired, inerrant and true Word of God: if part is true, all is true. If all of God's word is true, we must face the truth about our own moral character. Thus, through independent research and with the goal of Scripture proving Scripture rather than relying on what man says about God's Word, this book gradually came together exploring such topics as: what God says, statistical proof, historical and archeological evidence, and prophecy. And finally, we look at how the various versions of the Bible came about and a candid discussion is provided on how accurate or inaccurate they today's Bibles are. Let Dr. West-Stellick lead you on an exciting journal that lays the foundation, and then covers 3,500 years of writing, translations, discoveries leading to the you to the fact-based conclusion: The Bible IS God's Word to us. ISBN: 978-1887219105

In Sickness and in Health
In Sickness and in Health represents raw emotion. Inside you will find friends who have experienced what happens when chronic illness becomes the uninvited third member in your marital relationship. Inside, patients share their stories of pain and regret; partners and spouses share their frustrations, and fears. Both share the experiences of unplanned changes to their relationship. All share stories that are all too common when people gloss over the "In Sickness and in Health" part of their wedding vows, and reality sets in when someone is diagnosed with a life-altering chronic illness. This book provides a key message to all patients and partners: you are not alone. Others have walked (or been wheeled) in your shoes. *In Sickness and in Health*

provides the unique ability to learn what your partner is likely to be thinking and why he or she is behaving in a specific way that you may not know about. This book does not promise to transform your relationship, but it does promise to leave you with the knowledge that you are not alone in your journey. ISBN: 978-1887219204

God, Marriage, and Illness
It is a sobering truth. The divorce rate for physically healthy couples is between 40-50 %, the divorce rate for those plagued by chronic illness is in excess of 75 percent. When illness strikes, suddenly most people wonder what happened to that wonderful, caring, sensitive person they fell in love with. They wonder why they feel alone, and why they hurt even though they are still married or in a significant relationship. They wonder why their Godly marriage is falling apart. Part of the problem is focus. When there is a lack of reliance on God once illness presents in a marriage, the Illness, Marriage, and God paradigm needs to be transformed into one that places God first, followed by your marriage, and then, and only then, the focus on illness should enter into the triad. With the rate of chronic illnesses increasing at an alarming rate, readers must take action and INVEST to protect or repair their marriage in only the way that dependence and a focus on God can provide! What *God, Marriage, and Illness* offers is an interactive workbook designed to enable the reader a way to regain the proper perspective and focus on God first in their life.
ISBN: 978-188721920242

The God Prescription
Despite professional medical evidence that stresses prayer and attention to the spiritual life of a chronically ill patient dramatically serves to improve their quality of

life, upwards of 72% of all healthcare professionals never broach the subject with their patients, opting to focus instead on the medical model of patient care. Sadly, the traditional medical model draws the patient's attention away from the spiritual Godly realm and focuses it on the patient themselves. The real focus need to remain on Him, not the self. *The God Prescription* puts the focus back on God. *The God Prescription* can help you to: 1. Enhance your quality of life; 2. Reduce chronic pain and inflammation; 3. Transform limitations into opportunities that glorify God; and 4. Draw you closer to God. Writing from personal experience as a doctor and as a patient, Dr. West brings you: *The God Prescription.* ISBN: 978-1887219020

Fear of Forgetting Jesus
The Christian edition of *Fear of Forgetting*, delves into the heart and soul of a person diagnosed with Alzheimer's disease or one of the dementias as virtually every area of their Christian life is examined. Following a detailed presentation of the physiology involved in the disease progression, with the help of Scripture, areas of the individual's life are examined along with probing questions requiring the patient to document their feelings and experiences, along with their questions regarding risks, how they feel about memory loss and issues related to making new memories, including a major section delving into who the patient thinks Jesus is, their relationship with Jesus, familial history and experiences, favorite prayers, favorite Scriptures, and more. Like *Fear of Forgetting, Fear of Forgetting Jesus* guides the reader past their diagnosis and provides important information in an easy to understand way that educates the patient about what is really happening to their brain, what the journey will be like, and what they

can do about their diagnosis to embrace their journey. *Fear of Forgetting Jesus* is also purposely designed to enable easy reading for the older individual already in the early stages of the disease; in workbook format, it guides the patient through an introspective process of examining and documenting their fears, thoughts, and emotions about the diagnosis, the journey they will take, and *how they believe it will be best to reach them* as the disease progresses based on their unique life events, likes, and dislike, and should become a living journal for family and friends to use as a non-threatening springboard for discussion and care. And like *Fear of Forgetting, Fear of Forgetting Jesus* also includes the free bonus: *My Life, My Memories*, a special memory prompting diary all about who you are!
ISBN: 978-1887219273

My Life, My Memories
My Life, My Memories is a journal for completion by the dementia patient This journal will prompt you to write out answers to questions about your life, and your memories. The goal is to achieve a comprehensive book of your life, who you are, and what you are most likely to remember most as Alzheimer's disease or one of the other dementias progress. This journal will tie the patient's current life and past (stored memories) together. It will also help others to work with the patient in the later stages of the disease when, based on the patient's responses to the prompts in this book, for example, when you state likes and dislikes not only from the present but from the past. Topics covered include general information, work history, education, romance, childhood and teen years, religion, food, and a section where the patient can enter anything else that may have been overlooked but is considered by the patient to be

important! ISBN: 978-1887219327

Remembering Him Despite Dementia

Remembering Him Despite Dementia is essentially a follow-up book to Fear of Forgetting Jesus. When dementia strikes, although the brain cognitive and memory functions are gradually lost, our emotional attachments and connections remain virtually, up until the end. *Remembering Him Despite* Dementia focuses on the emotional attachments we have with the LORD. Whether they are from when one wasn't a believer, or whether they have been a believer all of their life, emphasizing the need to strengthen our emotional attachments to Christ can help those suffering from varied stages of dementia remain strong and resolute in Him. This will allow us to truly fill our hearts to overflowing for the LORD and overcome any fear of forgetting Jesus as dementia ravages our memory. ISBN: 978-1887219303

Paleo Basics: A delicious guide to what Paleo is all about, and how to become a Paleo Pro in no time!

Paleo Basics: A delicious guide to what Paleo is all about, and how to become a Paleo Pro in no time! is designed to provide a wealth of information on the why's and how-to's of starting on the Paleo Diet, filling in many of the gaps left in other books. For example, in Part One, *Paleo Basics* starts out explaining what the Paleo Diet is, and why a person should follow it, then goes on to discuss the finer points one needs to know in order to really make the Paleo Diet a lifestyle change. For example, setting up the Paleo kitchen, what is a Paleo grocery list like and how to construct one, how to grocery shop, and so forth. Then we talk about how to maintain a social life and remain on the Paleo Diet. Part Two picks up with super easy, delicious, and versatile recipes ranging from appetizers and breakfast dishes to sauces, snacks, and baked goods. This book is a must have to answer all the most common questions about going Paleo, and more than that, guides you through easy Paleo recipes that will ensure you can become a Paleo Pro in no time at all! ISBN: 978-1887219471

Paleo-licious Pasta! The definitive Paleo Pasta cookbook

Paleo-licious Pasta can give back the joy of pasta to those believed that following the Paleo diet completely removed that from the realm of pasta-bility! Part One details 10 different pasta recipes, ranging from the how-to's of making basic noodles to going beyond the basics with recipes for beet, tomato, spinach, and butternut squash pastas. Part Two provides over 50 exciting Paleo pasta recipes ranging from Paleo Mac N'Cheese to Turkey Tetrazzini. There's even a section on dessert pasta, including Paleo chocolate pasta in custard sauce, sweet Paleo noodle pudding, and Paleo strawberry pasta in lemon custard. ISBN: 978-1887219488

Consultations provided worldwide via Skype.

Please leave a message on my Facebook page link below:

Be sure to LIKE us on Facebook:
https://www.facebook.com/Alternatives-Naturopathy-101638931497584

All publications are available on Amazon throughout the world!

Made in the USA
Middletown, DE
06 July 2023

34648505R00060